PLANT- BASED COOKBOOK FOR TYPE 2 DIABETES

QUICK AND EASY RECIPES TO MANAGE AND CONTROL BLOOD SUGAR LEVEL IN NEWLY DIAGNOSED

HERRIENTA LAWSON

TABLE OF CONTENT

INTRODUCTION

A chronic illness that affects millions of people globally is type 2 diabetes. It is characterized by high blood sugar levels and can lead to serious health complications if left unmanaged. One of the most effective ways to manage and control blood sugar levels is through diet and lifestyle changes.

A plant-based diet has been shown to be not only beneficial for overall health but also effective in managing and controlling blood sugar levels in people with type 2 diabetes.

The Plant-Base Cookbook for Type 2 Diabetes: Quick and Easy Recipes to Manage and Control Blood Sugar Level in Newly Diagnosed is a comprehensive guide that offers delicious and nutritious plant-based recipes specifically designed for those with type 2 diabetes. Whether you have just been diagnosed or have been living with diabetes for years, this cookbook provides you with the tools and recipes you need to take control of your health and manage your blood sugar levels.

The cookbook starts with an introduction to type 2 diabetes and the importance of diet in managing the condition. It explains the principles of a plant-based diet and the benefits it provides for people with diabetes. The book also provides a basic overview of the essential nutrients and dietary guidelines needed to maintain stable blood sugar levels.

The recipes in the cookbook are quick and easy to prepare, making them perfect for those with busy lifestyles. Each recipe is carefully crafted to include a balance of carbohydrates, proteins, and healthy fats, ensuring that you get all the necessary nutrients while keeping your blood sugar levels in check.

The cookbook is divided into different sections, including breakfast, lunch, dinner, and snacks. There are also sections dedicated to desserts and beverages, so you can still enjoy some of your favorite treats without compromising your blood sugar levels. The recipes are accompanied by beautiful full-color photographs, making it easy to visualize the finished dish and get inspired to try new recipes.

Some of the delicious recipes you'll find in the cookbook include:

- **Oatmeal Breakfast Bowl:** A hearty and satisfying breakfast option packed with fiber and healthy grains to keep you full and energized throughout the morning.

- **Quinoa Salad with Roasted Vegetables:** A flavorful and nutrient-dense lunch option that combines roasted vegetables with protein-rich quinoa for a satisfying meal.

- **Chickpea Curry:** A flavorful dinner option that is rich in plant-based protein and packed with spices that have been shown to improve blood sugar control.

- **Avocado Chocolate Mousse:** A guilt-free dessert option that is creamy and indulgent, yet low in sugar and high in healthy fats.

- Green Smoothie: A refreshing and nutrient-packed beverage option that is perfect for a quick and healthy snack or breakfast on the go.

Each recipe in the cookbook includes detailed nutritional information, including the total carbohydrates, fiber, protein, and fat content, as well as the estimated glycemic index. This information is crucial for individuals with diabetes who need to monitor their carbohydrate intake, as carbohydrates have the greatest impact on blood sugar levels.

In addition to the recipes, the cookbook also provides valuable tips and suggestions for meal planning, grocery shopping, and navigating social situations while following a plant-based diet for diabetes. It also includes a two-week meal plan that can help you get started and provides guidance on portion sizes and meal timing.

Whether you're newly diagnosed with type 2 diabetes or have been living with the condition for years, the Plant Base Cookbook for Type 2 Diabetes is an essential resource for managing and controlling blood sugar levels through diet. With its delicious and easy-to-prepare recipes, helpful nutritional information, and practical tips, this cookbook will empower you to take control of your health and enjoy a variety of flavorful and satisfying meals while managing your blood sugar levels effectively. So why wait? Start your journey towards a healthier and happier life with the Type 2 Diabetic Plant-Based Diet Cookbook.

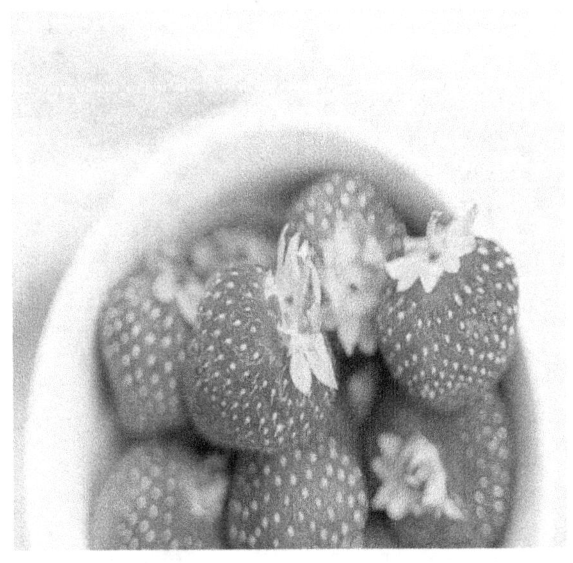

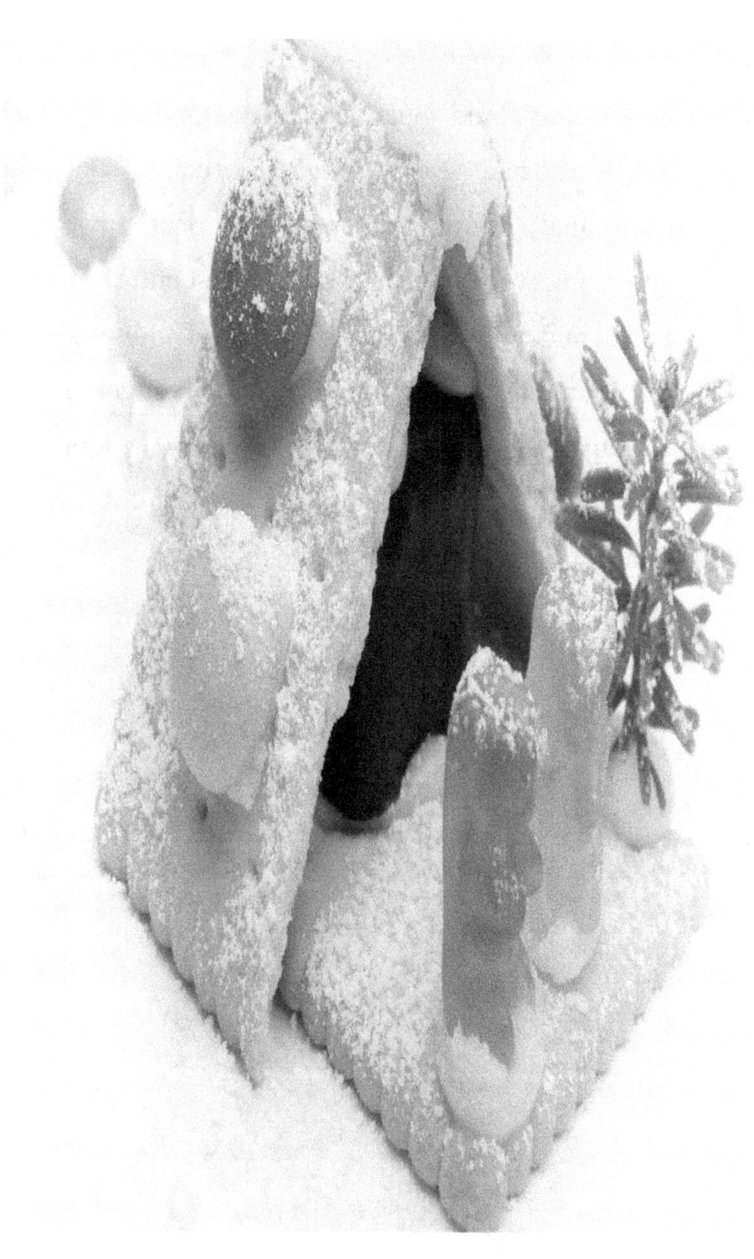

CHAPTER 1

Understanding type 2 diabetes and its dietary implications

1.1 What is type 2 diabetes?

Type 2 diabetes is a chronic metabolic disorder that affects how the body processes glucose (sugar). This condition occurs when the body becomes resistant to the effects of insulin, a hormone responsible for regulating blood sugar levels. As a result, the pancreas may produce insufficient amounts of insulin or the insulin produced is ineffective.

Poor diet, physical inactivity, and obesity are among the lifestyle variables that are frequently linked to type 2 diabetes.. It usually develops gradually over time and is more common in adults, while kids and teenagers may also be impacted.

The main characteristic of type 2 diabetes is high blood sugar levels, known as hyperglycemia. Symptoms may include frequent urination, excessive thirst, unexplained weight loss, increased hunger, fatigue, slow wound healing, and blurred vision. Some people, meanwhile, might not exhibit any obvious signs.

If left uncontrolled, type 2 diabetes can lead to serious complications such as heart disease, stroke, kidney damage, nerve damage, eye problems (retinopathy), and foot problems.

Treatment for type 2 diabetes involves making lifestyle changes such as adopting a healthy diet, engaging in regular physical activity, and maintaining a healthy weight. Medications may also be prescribed to control blood sugar levels, and in some cases, insulin therapy may be necessary to regulate blood glucose. Regular monitoring of blood sugar levels and regular check-ups with a healthcare provider are important for managing and controlling the condition.

The exact cause of type 2 diabetes is not fully understood, but it is believed to be a combination of genetic and environmental factors. Risk factors include being overweight or obese, leading a sedentary lifestyle, having a family history of diabetes, being over the age of 45, and certain ethnicities such as African-American, Hispanic, Native American, or Asian.

Insulin resistance: Insulin resistance is the main factor that defines type 2 diabetes. In insulin resistance, the body's cells become resistant to the effects of insulin, preventing glucose from entering the cells efficiently. This leads to a buildup of sugar in the bloodstream.

Insufficient insulin production: In addition to insulin resistance, type 2 diabetes can also involve the inadequate production of insulin by the pancreas. As the disease progresses, the pancreas may become less able to produce enough insulin to overcome insulin resistance. This further contributes to higher blood sugar levels.

Symptoms: Some common symptoms of type 2 diabetes include increased thirst, frequent urination (especially at night), unexplained weight loss, increased hunger, fatigue, blurred vision, slow wound healing, and frequent infections. However, some individuals may have no symptoms or only experience mild symptoms, which can make the diagnosis challenging. It's critical to recognize these signs and get medical assistance if they materialize.

Diagnosis: Type 2 diabetes is typically diagnosed through blood tests that measure fasting plasma glucose (FPG) levels or oral glucose tolerance tests (OGTT). A diagnosis is generally made if FPG levels are 126 mg/dL or higher, or if OGTT results show a blood sugar level of 200 mg/dL or higher after two hours.

Complications: If left untreated or poorly managed, type 2 diabetes can lead to several complications. These can include heart disease, stroke, kidney disease, nerve damage (neuropathy), eye damage (diabetic retinopathy), foot problems (diabetic neuropathy), and skin conditions. It is crucial to control blood sugar levels and manage the condition to help prevent these complications.

Treatment: Treatment for type 2 diabetes involves a multi-faceted approach. Lifestyle modifications are essential and include adopting a healthy diet, exercising regularly, losing weight if overweight, and quitting smoking if applicable. Medications may also be prescribed, including oral medications that help lower blood sugar levels or injections of insulin. Monitoring blood sugar levels regularly is important to track progress and adjust treatment accordingly. Additionally, patients with type 2 diabetes should receive regular check-ups with healthcare professionals to monitor their condition and manage any potential complications.

In summary, type 2 diabetes is a chronic condition characterized by insulin resistance and insufficient insulin production, resulting in high blood sugar levels. The main causes of it are a confluence of lifestyle and genetic variables. Diagnosis is made through blood tests, and treatment involves lifestyle modifications, medication, and regular monitoring to prevent complications.

1.2 The role of diet in type 2 diabetes management

One of the most important aspects of managing type 2 diabetes is diet. Type 2 diabetes is a condition characterized by high blood sugar levels, and diet can directly impact blood sugar levels and the body's ability to regulate insulin.

Here are some key ways in which diet can be beneficial in managing type 2 diabetes:

1. Controlling carbohydrate intake: Carbohydrates are broken down into glucose, which raises blood sugar levels. Therefore, monitoring and controlling carbohydrate intake is essential for managing blood sugar levels. This can be done by choosing complex carbohydrates over simple carbohydrates, including whole grains, fruits, vegetables, legumes, and avoiding refined sugars and processed foods.

2. Balancing meals: Eating regular and balanced meals throughout the day can help in managing blood sugar levels. It is recommended to include a variety of macronutrients (carbohydrates, proteins, and fats) in each meal as it can slow down the absorption of glucose into the bloodstream.

3. Portion control: Managing portion sizes is vital for individuals with type 2 diabetes. Overeating can lead to elevated blood sugar levels, weight gain, and insulin resistance. Monitoring portion sizes and eating mindfully can help in maintaining a healthy weight and managing blood sugar levels.

4. Choosing healthy fats: Including healthy fats such as olive oil, avocados, nuts, and seeds in the diet can help in managing blood sugar levels. These fats are known to have a positive effect on insulin sensitivity and can help in reducing inflammation.

5. Increasing fiber intake: Fiber has numerous benefits for individuals with type 2 diabetes. It helps regulate blood sugar levels by slowing down the absorption of glucose and improving insulin sensitivity. Including high-fiber foods such as whole grains, fruits, vegetables, legumes, and nuts can be beneficial.

6. Limiting processed and sugary foods: Processed and sugary foods are often high in refined carbohydrates and unhealthy fats. These foods can lead to spikes in blood sugar levels and can contribute to weight gain. It is important to limit the consumption of sugary beverages, desserts, processed snacks, and sweetened cereals.

7. Regular monitoring and guidance: It is crucial for individuals with type 2 diabetes to regularly monitor their blood sugar levels and work closely with healthcare providers, including registered dietitians, to develop personalized meal plans and make necessary adjustments. Healthcare professionals can provide guidance and support in understanding nutritional labels, carbohydrate counting, and implementing an individualized eating plan.

While diet is an important component of managing type 2 diabetes, it is essential to note that individualized care and lifestyle modifications should be tailored to each person's unique needs and preferences. It is recommended to consult with healthcare professionals for personalized advice and guidance in managing type 2 diabetes through diet.

Overall, diet plays a crucial role in the management of type 2 diabetes. By controlling carbohydrate intake, balancing meals, practicing portion control, choosing healthy fats, increasing fiber intake, limiting processed and sugary foods, and receiving regular monitoring and guidance, individuals with type 2 diabetes can effectively manage their blood sugar levels and improve overall health. It is important to work closely with healthcare professionals to develop a personalized eating plan that fits individual needs, preferences, and lifestyle.

A plant-based diet has several benefits for blood sugar control. These are a handful of the principal benefits:

1. Low glycemic index: Plant-based foods tend to have a lower glycemic index compared to animal-based foods. This means they have a slower and steadier effect on blood sugar levels, preventing spikes and crashes that can occur with high-glycemic foods.

2. High in fiber: Plant-based foods are typically high in dietary fiber, which slows down the absorption of glucose into the bloodstream. This lessens the chance of unexpected surges in blood sugar levels.

3. Rich in complex carbohydrates: Complex carbohydrates found in plant-based foods take longer to break down into glucose compared to simple carbohydrates found in processed foods.

This slower digestion process helps to stabilize blood sugar levels and provide a sustained release of energy.

4. Nutrient-dense: Plant-based diets are typically rich in vitamins, minerals, and antioxidants, which can help improve insulin sensitivity and reduce the risk of developing type 2 diabetes. These nutrients also support overall health and well-being.

5. Lower in saturated fat and cholesterol: Animal-based foods, such as meat and dairy products, are often high in saturated fat and cholesterol. Consuming a plant-based diet can help reduce the intake of these unhealthy fats, which can improve insulin sensitivity and reduce the risk of insulin resistance and type 2 diabetes.

6. Weight management: Plant-based diets are generally lower in calories and higher in fiber, which can aid in weight management. Maintaining a healthy weight is important for blood sugar control, as excess body weight can contribute to insulin resistance and diabetes.

7. Reduced inflammation: Plant-based diets are known to have anti-inflammatory properties due to their high content of antioxidants and phytonutrients. This can help reduce chronic inflammation, which is associated with insulin resistance and diabetes.

8. Lower risk of cardiovascular disease: Plant-based diets are associated with a lower risk of cardiovascular disease, which is a common complication of diabetes. By reducing the risk of heart disease, a plant-based diet can help individuals with diabetes improve their overall health and reduce their risk of cardiovascular complications.

9. Improved gut health: Plant-based diets are typically high in prebiotic fibers, which promote the growth of beneficial gut bacteria. A healthy gut microbiome is crucial for blood sugar control, as it affects the digestion and absorption of carbohydrates, as well as insulin sensitivity.

10. Sustainable lifestyle: In addition to blood sugar control and health benefits, a plant-based diet is also more sustainable and environmentally friendly than a diet that includes animal products. Animal agriculture is a major contributor to greenhouse gas emissions, deforestation, and water pollution. By adopting a plant-based diet, individuals can reduce their environmental impact and contribute to a more sustainable future.

Overall, a plant-based diet offers numerous benefits for blood sugar control, including improved glycemic control, weight management, reduced inflammation, and a lower risk of cardiovascular disease and type 2 diabetes. It is a nutritious and sustainable dietary approach that can support overall health and well-being.

Additionally, a plant-based diet is rich in antioxidants and phytochemicals that can help reduce oxidative stress and inflammation in the body. Chronic inflammation is a known contributor to insulin resistance and high blood sugar levels, so consuming a plant-based diet can help reduce the risk of developing these conditions.

Furthermore, a plant-based diet is naturally low in saturated fats and cholesterol, which are found in high amounts in animal-based foods. High intake of saturated fats and cholesterol has been linked to insulin resistance and an increased risk of developing type 2 diabetes. By choosing plant-based sources of protein, such as legumes, tofu, or tempeh, individuals can maintain a healthy blood lipid profile and improve their insulin sensitivity.

Moreover, a plant-based diet is high in dietary fiber, which is crucial for blood sugar control. Carbohydrate digestion and absorption are slowed down by fiber, which helps to delay sharp rises in blood sugar. It also promotes a feeling of fullness, helping individuals maintain a healthy weight and prevent overeating.

Lastly, a plant-based diet can positively impact overall cardiovascular health. High blood sugar levels increase the risk of cardiovascular disease, and individuals with diabetes are at a higher risk of developing heart disease. By adopting a plant-based diet, individuals can improve their blood sugar control, lower their blood pressure and cholesterol levels, and reduce their risk of developing heart disease.

In conclusion, a plant-based diet offers numerous benefits for blood sugar control. It is rich in nutrients, high in fiber, low in saturated fats, and can help reduce inflammation and oxidative stress in the body. By adopting a plant-based diet, individuals can improve their insulin sensitivity, regulate their blood sugar levels, reduce their risk of developing type 2 diabetes, and promote overall cardiovascular health.

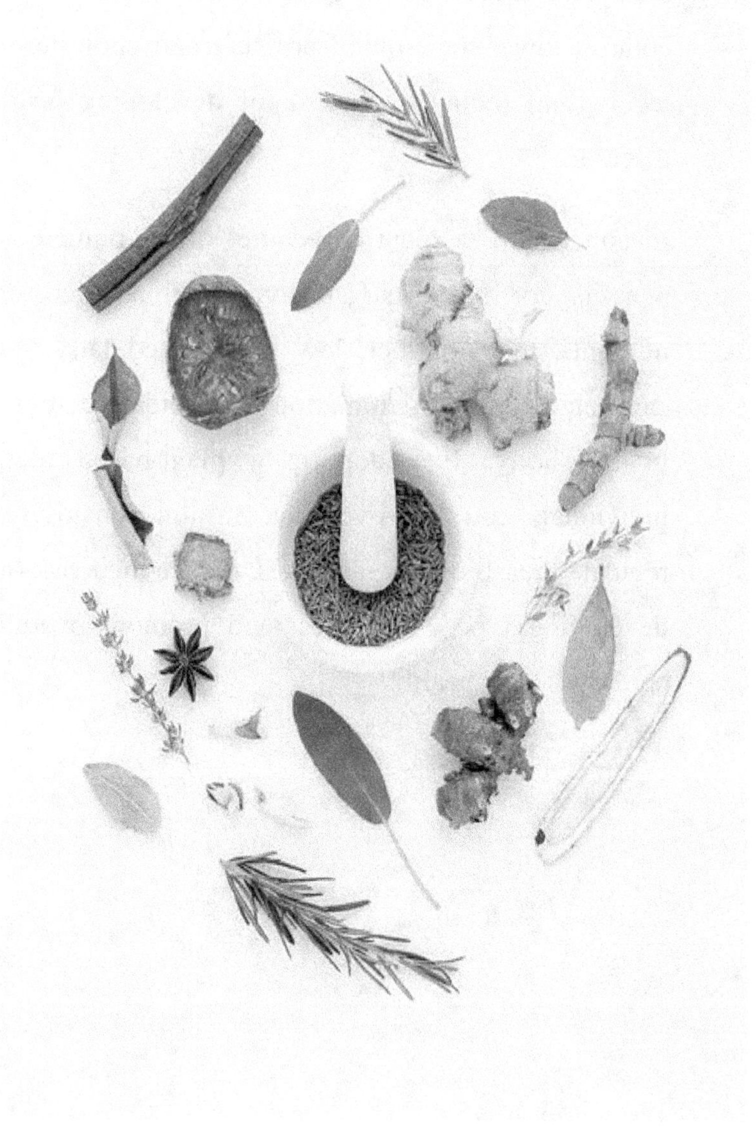

CHAPTER 2

Getting started with a plant-based diet for type 2 diabetes

2.1 transitioning to a plant-based lifestyle

Transitioning to a plant-based lifestyle can have numerous benefits for individuals with type 2 diabetes. Adopting a diet rich in fruits, vegetables, whole grains, legumes, and plant-based proteins can help manage blood sugar levels, improve heart health, and promote overall well-being.

One of the key advantages of a plant-based diet for individuals with type 2 diabetes is its ability to support weight loss and weight management. Plants are typically low in calories and high in fiber, which helps promote satiety and can lead to a reduced calorie intake. By shedding excess weight, individuals can improve insulin sensitivity and better manage their blood sugar levels.

Moreover, plant-based diets are naturally low in saturated fats and cholesterol, which can contribute to heart disease. By reducing or eliminating the consumption of animal products, individuals can decrease their risk of developing cardiovascular complications, which frequently accompany type 2 diabetes.

Focusing on whole, unprocessed foods can also improve glycemic control. Whole grains, such as brown rice, quinoa, and whole wheat bread, have a lower glycemic index compared to their refined counterparts. This means they are digested more slowly, resulting in a slower release of glucose into the bloodstream and therefore better blood sugar control.

Additionally, plant-based diets are rich in fiber, which helps slow down the digestion and absorption of carbohydrates. This leads to a more gradual rise in blood sugar levels after meals, reducing the risk of spikes and crashes. Fiber has also been shown to improve insulin sensitivity and reduce insulin resistance, making it easier for the body to regulate blood sugar.

Plant-based diets are also abundant in antioxidants, vitamins, and minerals, which can help reduce inflammation and oxidative stress – two common factors associated with type 2 diabetes. By incorporating a variety of colorful fruits and vegetables into your diet, you can provide your body with essential nutrients that support overall health and well-being.

When transitioning to a plant-based lifestyle for type 2 diabetes, it's important to consult with a healthcare professional, such as a registered dietitian or nutritionist, to ensure a balanced and nutritious diet. They can help you determine appropriate portion sizes, recommend specific foods to include in your diet, and ensure you are meeting your nutritional needs.

It's also essential to gradually make changes to your diet, as sudden and drastic changes may be difficult to sustain. Start by adding more fruits, vegetables, and plant-based proteins to your meals, and gradually decrease your consumption of animal products. Experiment with new recipes, flavors, and cooking methods to make your plant-based meals more enjoyable and satisfying.

Finally, adopting a plant-based lifestyle can have positive effects beyond managing type 2 diabetes. It can help lower blood pressure, reduce the risk of developing certain cancers, improve digestion, and support weight management. It is important to remember that everyone's dietary needs and preferences may vary, and it's essential to listen to your body and make choices that work best for you.

In conclusion, transitioning to a plant-based lifestyle can be a highly beneficial approach for individuals with type 2 diabetes. By focusing on whole, unprocessed plant foods, reducing the intake of animal products, and incorporating a variety of fruits, vegetables, whole grains, and legumes, individuals can improve blood sugar control, manage weight, and promote overall health.

Consulting with a healthcare professional and taking a gradual approach can help ensure a successful transition to a plant-based diet that meets your nutritional needs and supports your journey towards a healthier lifestyle.

2.2 Essential pantry staples for a diabetic-friendly plant-based diet

If you have diabetes and are following a plant-based diet, it's important to stock your pantry with the right foods to help you maintain stable blood sugar levels and meet your dietary needs. Here are some essential pantry staples for a diabetic-friendly plant-based diet:

1. Legumes: Lentils, chickpeas, black beans, and other legumes are excellent sources of plant-based protein and complex carbohydrates. They are also high in fiber, which helps regulate blood sugar levels. Canned or dry legumes are both good options, but if you opt for canned, choose low-sodium varieties and rinse them well before use.

2. Whole grains: Switching to whole grains like brown rice, quinoa, oats, and whole wheat pasta can provide more fiber and nutrients compared to refined grains. They digest more slowly, which can prevent blood sugar spikes. Brown rice can be an excellent alternative to white rice as it has a lower glycemic index.

3. Nuts and seeds: Almonds, walnuts, flaxseeds, and chia seeds are great sources of healthy fats, protein, and fiber. They can help keep you feeling full and satisfied, which is important for managing hunger and preventing overeating.

4. Non-dairy milk: Options like almond milk, soy milk, and oat milk make great alternatives to cow's milk for those following a plant-based diet. Seek unsweetened types to stay away from ones with extra sugar. These milks also provide essential nutrients such as calcium and vitamin D.

5. Healthy fats: Include sources of healthy fats in your pantry, such as avocado oil, olive oil, and coconut oil. These fats can help improve insulin sensitivity and provide satiety. Use them in moderation and opt for extra virgin or cold-pressed oils whenever possible.

6. Herbs and spices: Flavoring your meals with herbs and spices instead of using excessive salt or sugar can help you reduce sodium and manage blood pressure. Stock your pantry with various herbs like basil, oregano, thyme, and spices like cinnamon, turmeric, cumin, and paprika.

7. Low-sodium sauces and condiments: Choose sugar-free, low-sodium sauces and condiments to add flavor to your meals. Look for options like low-sodium soy sauce, balsamic vinegar, mustard, and salsa. These alternatives can enhance the taste of your food without adding unnecessary sodium or added sugars.

8. Unsweetened applesauce: Unsweetened applesauce can be used in baking recipes as a substitute for oil or sugar. It adds natural sweetness and moisture to your dishes without negatively impacting your blood sugar levels.

9. Canned or jarred tomatoes: Canned or jarred tomatoes are a convenient option to have in your pantry. They can be used as a base for sauces, soups, and stews, providing a healthy dose of lycopene, vitamins, and minerals. Look for no-salt-added options to control your sodium intake.

10. Sugar substitutes: If you need to sweeten your dishes, opt for natural sugar substitutes like stevia, monk fruit, or erythritol. These options have minimal impact on blood sugar levels and can be used in moderation as a substitute for refined sugars.

Remember to check food labels and opt for low-sodium, low-sugar, and whole food-based options whenever possible. By keeping your pantry stocked with these essential staples, you can ensure you have plenty of nutritious options on hand for a diabetic-friendly plant-based diet.

Meal Planning and Preparing for Success for Type 2 Diabetes Plant-Based Diet

1. Start with a grocery list: Plan your meals for the week and create a detailed grocery list before you head to the store. Include a variety of fruits, vegetables, whole grains, legumes, and plant-based proteins to ensure a well-balanced diet.

2. Stay hydrated: Water is essential for overall health and helps regulate blood sugar levels. Make sure to drink enough water throughout the day, and limit sugary drinks and alcohol.

3. Focus on whole foods: Fill your plate with whole, unprocessed foods such as vegetables, fruits, whole grains, legumes, and nuts. These provide nutrients, fiber, and antioxidants that can help manage blood sugar levels.

4. Get creative with plant-based protein sources: Incorporate a variety of plant-based protein sources into your meals, such as tofu, tempeh, lentils, beans, and chickpeas. These foods are not only rich in protein but also contain fiber, which can help stabilize blood sugar levels.

5. Include healthy fats: Opt for healthy fats like avocado, nuts, and seeds in your meals. These fats are rich in omega-3 fatty acids, which have been shown to improve insulin sensitivity and reduce inflammation.

6. Control portion sizes: Pay attention to portion sizes to avoid overeating and help manage blood sugar levels. Use smaller plates and bowls, and aim to fill half of your plate with non-starchy vegetables, one-quarter with whole grains or starchy vegetables, and one-quarter with plant-based protein.

7. Meal prep in advance: Set aside time each week to meal prep and batch cook your meals. This will save you time and ensure that you have healthy, plant-based meals readily available when you're feeling hungry or pressed for time.

8. Choose low glycemic index foods: Opt for foods with a low glycemic index (GI), which means they have a slower impact on blood sugar levels. These consist of most fruits, whole grains, legumes, and non-starchy vegetables. These consist of most fruits, whole grains, legumes, and non-starchy vegetables.

9. Experiment with spices and herbs: Use herbs and spices to add flavor to your meals instead of relying on excessive amounts of salt or sugar. Experiment with different combinations to create delicious and satisfying dishes.

10. Monitor your blood sugar levels: Keep track of your blood sugar levels regularly to see how your diet affects them. This will help you fine-tune your meal planning and make adjustments if needed.

Remember, it's important to consult with a healthcare professional or registered dietitian before making any significant changes to your diet, especially if you have type 2 diabetes. They can provide personalized recommendations and support to help you manage your blood sugar levels.

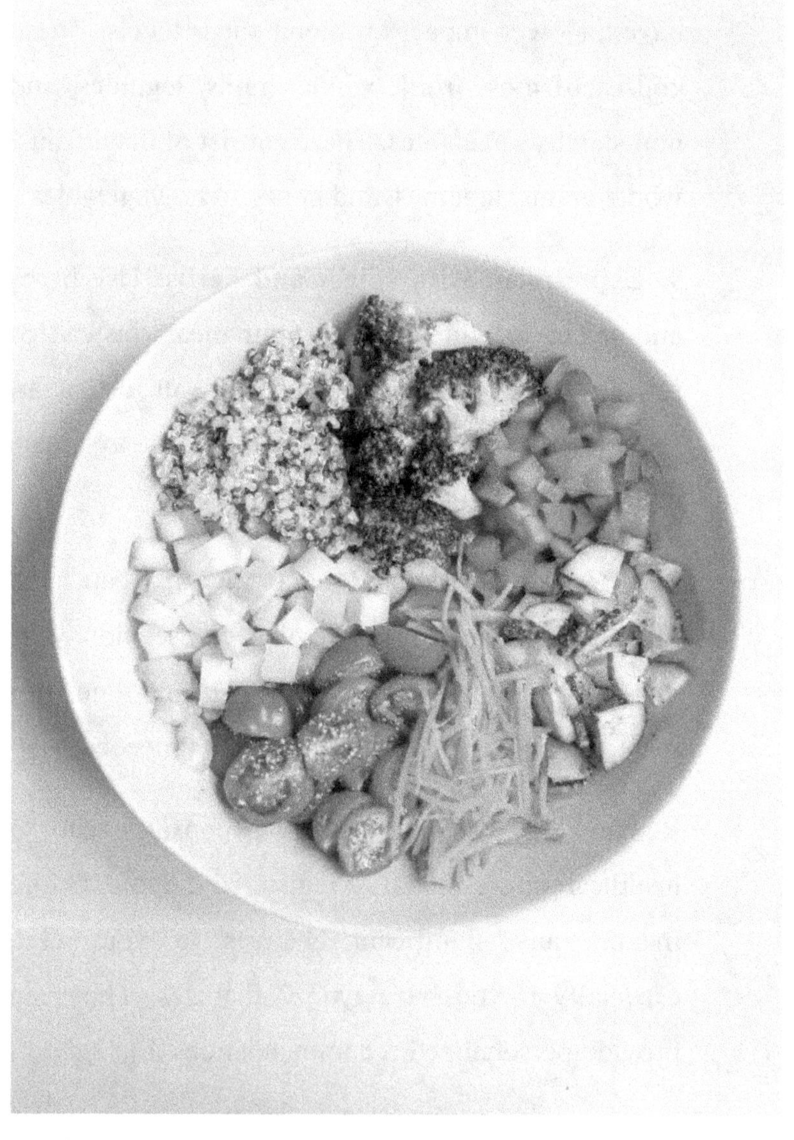

CHAPTER 3

Breakfast recipes to kick start your day

3.1 Easy overnight oats with berries

Overnight oats have become a popular breakfast choice for those who are seeking a quick and nutritious meal to kick-start their day. With just a little bit of preparation the night before, you can have a delicious and filling bowl of oats waiting for you in the morning. One of the best ways to enjoy overnight oats is by adding a variety of berries to amplify the flavor and nutritional value.

Here is a simple recipe for easy overnight oats with berries:

Ingredients:

- 1/2 cup rolled oats

- 1/2 cup milk (dairy or plant-based)

- 1/2 cup Greek yogurt

- 1 tablespoon chia seeds

- One tablespoon (optional) of maple syrup or honey

- 1/2 cup mixed berries (such as strawberries, blueberries, raspberries)

- A handful of nuts or granola for topping (optional)

Instructions:

1. In a jar or container with a lid, combine the rolled oats, milk, Greek yogurt, chia seeds, and sweetener (if desired). Stir well to combine all the ingredients.

2. Gently fold in the mixed berries, making sure they are evenly distributed throughout the mixture.

3. Cover the jar or container with a lid and place it in the refrigerator overnight, or for at least 4 hours. This allows the oats to soak up the liquid and become soft and creamy.

4. In the morning, give the oats a stir to incorporate the berries throughout. If the mixture seems too thick, you can add a splash of milk to loosen it up.

5. Serve the oats in a bowl and top with additional berries, nuts, or granola for added crunch and texture.

6. Enjoy your easy overnight oats with berries!

This recipe's easy customization is one of its many wonderful features. You can switch up the type of berries you use based on your preference or what's in season. You can also add other ingredients, such as sliced bananas, shredded coconut, or a sprinkle of cinnamon, for added flavor.

Berries are an excellent addition to overnight oats due to their natural sweetness and numerous health benefits. They are packed with antioxidants, vitamins, and fiber, making them a nutritious and delicious choice. They also add a burst of color and freshness to your breakfast bowl.

Not only are these overnight oats with berries simple to prepare, but they also make for a convenient on-the-go breakfast option. You can easily prepare them in advance and grab them in the morning as you rush out the door.

These easy overnight oats with berries are not only delicious but also provide you with a balanced and nutritious breakfast. They are a great source of protein, fiber, and healthy fats, which will keep you satisfied and energized throughout the morning.

So why not give this recipe a try? It's a quick and easy way to enjoy a wholesome and flavorful breakfast without much effort. Plus, with the addition of the vibrant and juicy berries, it will make your morning meal even more enjoyable. Give it a go and start your day on a healthy and tasty note!

3.2 Veggie-packed scramble

This recipe is perfect for those who want to incorporate more vegetables into their diet without sacrificing flavor.

To make this veggie-packed scramble, you will need the following ingredients:

- 2 tablespoons olive oil

- 1 small onion, diced

- 1 bell pepper, diced

- 1 zucchini, diced

- 1 cup mushrooms, sliced

- 2 cups baby spinach

- ½ teaspoon salt

- ½ teaspoon black pepper

- ½ teaspoon garlic powder

- 6 large eggs

- ¼ cup milk (optional)

- ½ cup shredded cheese of your choice (optional)

To begin, place a large skillet over medium heat with the olive oil.. Add the diced onion and sauté until it becomes translucent, about 2-3 minutes. Next, add in the diced bell pepper, zucchini, and sliced mushrooms. Cook the vegetables for about 5-7 minutes, or until they have softened.

Once the vegetables are cooked, add in the baby spinach and stir until it wilts. Season the mixture with salt, black pepper, and garlic powder, and give it a quick stir.

Whisk the eggs and milk together in a another basin. Pour the egg mixture into the skillet with the cooked vegetables, making sure to evenly distribute the mixture. Gently scramble the eggs with a spatula, stirring occasionally, until they are cooked to your desired consistency. The cooking time will vary depending on how soft or firm you prefer your eggs.

If desired, sprinkle shredded cheese over the scramble and cover the skillet for a minute to allow the cheese to melt. Once the cheese has melted, remove the skillet from the heat and serve the veggie-packed scramble immediately.

This recipe is incredibly versatile and can be customized to your taste preferences. Feel free to add any other vegetables you have on hand, such as cherry tomatoes, broccoli, or even grated carrots. To improve the flavor, try experimenting with other herbs and spices.

Serve the veggie-packed scramble as it is, or pair it with some whole grain toast, avocado slices, or a side of fresh fruit. This dish not only makes a satisfying breakfast, but it can also be enjoyed for brunch, lunch, or even a quick dinner.

With its vibrant colors and delicious flavors, this veggie-packed scramble is a great way to increase your vegetable intake and start your day on a healthy note.

Blueberry-Flaxseed Smoothie Bowl Recipe

Ingredients:

- 1 cup frozen blueberries

- 1 ripe banana

- 1 cup spinach or kale

- 1 tablespoon flaxseeds

- 1 tablespoon almond butter

- 1 cup unsweetened almond milk or any milk of your choice

- Toppings (optional): fresh blueberries, sliced bananas, shredded coconut, granola, chia seeds, or any other desired toppings

Instructions:

1. In a high-speed blender, combine the frozen blueberries, banana, spinach or kale, flaxseeds, almond butter, and almond milk.

2. Process on high speed until creamy and smooth. To get the right consistency, add more almond milk if the mixture is too thick.

3. Pour the smoothie into a bowl.

4. Decorate the smoothie bowl with your favorite toppings, such as fresh blueberries, sliced bananas, shredded coconut, granola, and chia seeds.

5. Enjoy your refreshing and nutritious blueberry-flaxseed smoothie bowl!

Benefits of Blueberry-Flaxseed Smoothie Bowl:

1. Blueberries are rich in antioxidants, which help fight free radicals and reduce inflammation in the body.

2. Flaxseeds are an excellent source of fiber and omega-3 fatty acids, which promote heart health and aid in digestion.

3. Spinach or kale adds essential vitamins and minerals, including iron and vitamin K, to support overall health.

4. Banana provides natural sweetness and adds potassium, which is beneficial for maintaining healthy blood pressure levels.

5. Almond butter offers a creamy texture and adds healthy fats and protein to keep you full and satisfied.

6. Unsweetened almond milk is a dairy-free and low-calorie option that provides calcium and vitamin D.

This delicious blueberry-flaxseed smoothie bowl is not only a treat for your taste buds but also a powerhouse of nutrients to start your day on a healthy note.

CHAPTER 4

Wholesome lunches for sustained energy

4.1 Mediterranean quinoa salad

Mediterranean Quinoa Salad is a refreshing and nutritious dish packed with Mediterranean flavors. It is a perfect option for a light lunch or a side dish for any meal. This recipe combines quinoa, fresh vegetables, feta cheese, and a tangy lemon dressing, creating a vibrant and satisfying salad.

Ingredients:

- 1 cup quinoa

- 2 cups water

- 1 cup cherry tomatoes, halved

- 1 cucumber, diced

- 1 red bell pepper, diced

- 1/2 red onion, thinly sliced

- Half a cup of Kalamata olives, pitted and cut in half

- 1/2 cup crumbled feta cheese

- 1/4 cup chopped fresh parsley

- 1/4 cup fresh lemon juice

- 2 tablespoons extra-virgin olive oil

- 2 garlic cloves, minced

- Salt and pepper to taste

Instructions:

1. Use a fine-mesh strainer to rinse and thoroughly drain the quinoa.

2. Place the water in a medium pot and bring it to a boil.

 Add the quinoa and a pinch of salt. Reduce the heat to low, cover, and simmer for about 15-20 minutes, or until all the water is absorbed and the quinoa is tender. Remove from heat and let it cool for a few minutes.

3. In a large mixing bowl, combine the cooked quinoa, cherry tomatoes, cucumber, red bell pepper, red onion, kalamata olives, feta cheese, and chopped parsley.

4. In a small bowl, whisk together the lemon juice, olive oil, minced garlic, salt, and pepper until well combined.

5. Pour the dressing over the quinoa mixture and toss gently until everything is evenly coated.

6. Taste and, if necessary, adjust seasoning.

7. Cover the bowl and refrigerate the salad for at least 30 minutes to allow thc flavors to meld together.

8. Serve chilled and garnish with additional fresh parsley if desired.

This Mediterranean Quinoa Salad can be customized to suit your taste. You can add or substitute ingredients such as roasted red peppers, artichoke hearts, chickpeas, or fresh basil leaves. It is a versatile and filling dish that can be enjoyed on its own or served alongside grilled chicken or fish. The tangy lemon dressing adds a bright and zesty flavor that complements the fresh vegetables and nutty quinoa.

4.2 Roasted sweet potato and chickpea buddha bowl

If you're looking for a healthy and filling meal, look no further than this roasted sweet potato and chickpea buddha bowl. Packed with flavor and nutrients, this colorful bowl is a perfect balance of carbohydrates, protein, and healthy fats. Plus, it's easy to customize with your favorite toppings and dressings.

Ingredients:

- One big sweet potato, chopped and skinned

- 1 can chickpeas, rinsed and drained

- 1 tablespoon olive oil

- 1 teaspoon paprika

- 1/2 teaspoon cumin

- 1/2 teaspoon garlic powder

- Salt and pepper, to taste

- 4 cups cooked quinoa or brown rice

- 2 cups fresh spinach

- 1 avocado, sliced

- 1/4 cup sliced almonds

- Optional toppings: cherry tomatoes, cucumber, feta cheese, tahini dressing, etc.

Instructions:

1. Preheat your oven to 400°F (200°C).

2. In a large mixing bowl, toss together the sweet potato, chickpeas, olive oil, paprika, cumin, garlic powder, salt, and pepper until evenly coated.

3. Spread the sweet potato and chickpea mixture onto a baking sheet lined with parchment paper.

4. Roast in the preheated oven for 25-30 minutes or until the sweet potatoes are tender and golden brown.

5. While the sweet potatoes and chickpeas are roasting, prepare your quinoa or brown rice according to package instructions.

6. Once the sweet potatoes and chickpeas are done, remove them from the oven and set aside to cool slightly.

7. Assemble your buddha bowl by dividing the cooked quinoa or brown rice into four serving bowls.

8. Top each bowl with a handful of fresh spinach, roasted sweet potatoes and chickpeas, sliced avocado, and sliced almonds.

9. Add any additional toppings of your choice such as cherry tomatoes, cucumber, feta cheese, or a drizzle of tahini dressing.

10. Serve immediately and enjoy your delicious and nutritious roasted sweet potato and chickpea buddha bowl.

This recipe is not only visually appealing but also offers a perfect combination of flavors and textures. The sweet potatoes add a natural sweetness while the chickpeas provide protein and fiber. The addition of fresh spinach gives a refreshing taste, and the avocado brings healthy fats to the dish. The sliced almonds add a nice crunch and a dose of healthy fats as well.

Feel free to customize this Buddha bowl to your liking. You can add other vegetables like cherry tomatoes or cucumber for extra freshness. If you prefer a creamier dressing, drizzle some tahini dressing over the bowl. And if you're a fan of cheese, sprinkle some crumbled feta on top for added richness.

Not only is this roasted sweet potato and chickpea Buddha bowl delicious, but it's also a wholesome and well-rounded meal. The combination of whole grains, protein, and vegetables makes it a satisfying option for lunch or dinner. Plus, it's easy to prep and perfect for meal prepping. Simply roast the sweet potatoes and chickpeas ahead of time, cook the quinoa or brown rice, and assemble the bowls when you're ready to eat.

Try this recipe for a satisfying and nourishing meal that will leave you feeling energized and satisfied.

4.3 Zucchini noodle stir-fry with tofu

Ingredients:

- 2 medium zucchini

- One firm tofu block, drained and sliced into cubes

- 2 tablespoons soy sauce

- 1 tablespoon sesame oil

- 1 tablespoon rice vinegar

- 1 tablespoon maple syrup (vegan variant) or honey

- 2 cloves garlic, minced

- 1 teaspoon ginger, grated

- 1 red bell pepper, thinly sliced

- 1 carrot, thinly sliced

- 1 cup broccoli florets

- 1 cup snap peas

- 2 green onions, chopped

- Sesame seeds, for garnish

- Salt and pepper, to taste

Instructions:

1. To make zucchini noodles, use a spiralizer or vegetable peeler to create long, thin noodles. Set aside. If you don't have a spiralizer, you can also use a julienne peeler or a knife to cut the zucchini into thin strips.

2. In a small bowl, whisk together soy sauce, sesame oil, rice vinegar, honey (or maple syrup), minced garlic, and grated ginger. Set aside.

3. Heat a large skillet or wok over medium-high heat. Add tofu cubes and cook until evenly brown on all sides. This should take about 5-7 minutes. Take out and place aside the tofu from the skillet.

4. In the same skillet, add the sliced bell pepper, carrot, broccoli, and snap peas. Stir-fry for about 3-4 minutes until the vegetables are slightly tender but still crisp.

5. Add the zucchini noodles to the skillet and stir-fry for an additional 2-3 minutes. You want to cook the zucchini noodles until they are just tender but still have a slight crunch.

6. Pour the sauce mixture over the zucchini noodles and vegetables. Stir well to coat everything evenly.

7. Add the cooked tofu back into the skillet and gently toss to combine.

8. Season with salt and pepper, to taste.

9. Turn off the heat and sprinkle with sesame seeds and finely chopped green onions.

10. Serve immediately and enjoy!

This zucchini noodle stir-fry with tofu is a healthy and delicious option for a quick weeknight meal. The zucchini noodles add a light and refreshing touch to the dish while the tofu provides a good source of plant-based protein. Feel free to customize the stir-fry with your favorite vegetables or add additional spices or sauces to suit your taste.

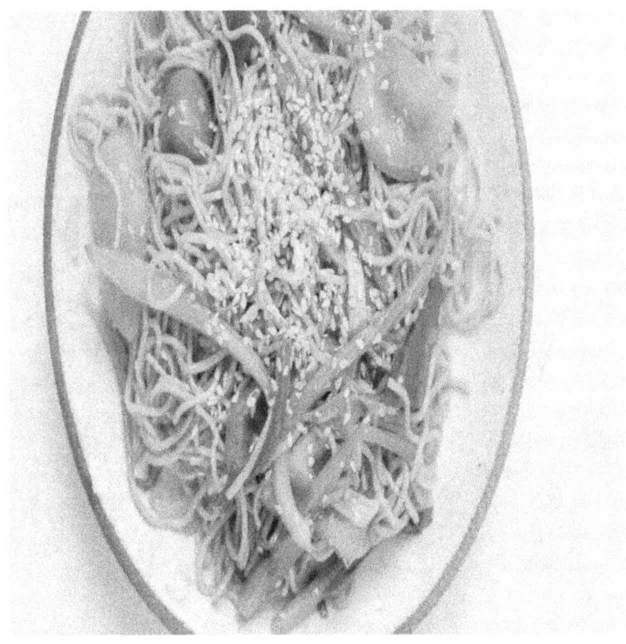

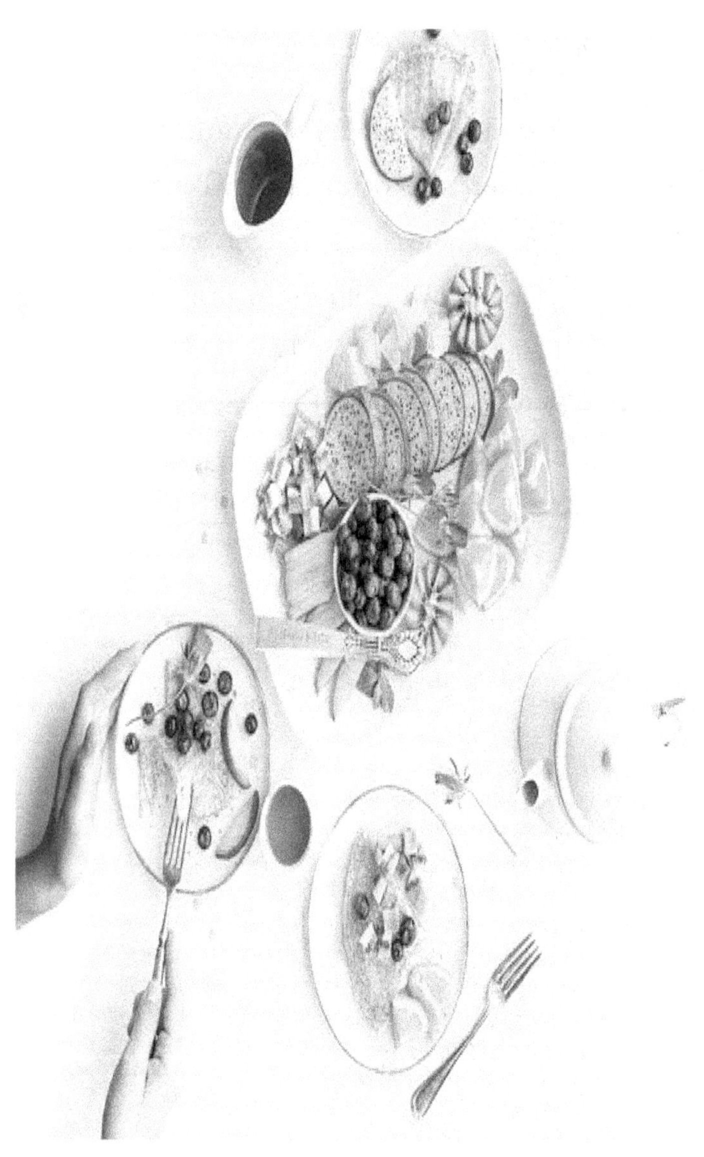

CHAPTER 5

5.1 Spicy black bean and corn tacos

Ingredients:

- 1 can black beans, drained and rinsed

- 1 cup frozen corn kernels

- 1 small red onion, diced

- 1 jalapeno pepper, seeded and diced

- 2 cloves garlic, minced

- 1 teaspoon ground cumin

- 1 teaspoon chili powder

- 1/2 teaspoon paprika

- 1/4 teaspoon cayenne pepper (optional, for extra spice)

- Salt and pepper to taste

- 8 small flour or corn tortillas

- Toppings: sliced avocado, chopped cilantro, crumbled queso fresco, lime wedges

Instructions:

1. Heat the olive oil in a big skillet over medium heat. Add diced red onion and jalapeno pepper, and sauté until softened, about 5 minutes.

2. Add minced garlic and spices (cumin, chili powder, paprika, cayenne pepper), and cook for another minute until aromatic.

3. Add black beans and corn to the skillet, stirring well to combine with the spices. Cook for about 5-7 minutes, until the beans and corn are heated through.

4. To taste, add salt and pepper for seasoning.

5. Meanwhile, heat a separate skillet or griddle over medium heat. Warm the tortillas on each side for a few seconds, until soft and pliable.

6. Assemble the tacos by spooning the black bean and corn mixture onto each tortilla. Top with sliced avocado, chopped cilantro, crumbled queso fresco, and a squeeze of lime juice.

7. Serve the spicy black bean and corn tacos hot and enjoy!

Note: You can customize these tacos by adding additional toppings such as salsa, sour cream, or hot sauce. You can also add some protein, like grilled chicken or shrimp, if desired. If you prefer a milder flavor, you can decrease the amount of spices or omit the cayenne pepper.

5.2 Lentil curry with cauliflower rice

Lentil Curry with Cauliflower Rice Recipe

If you're looking for a flavorful and healthy vegetarian dish, this Lentil Curry with Cauliflower Rice is the perfect choice. Packed with nutritious ingredients and aromatic spices, this dish is sure to satisfy your taste buds while keeping you feeling full and satisfied.

Ingredients:

For the Lentil Curry:

- 1 cup red lentils, rinsed

- 1 onion, diced

- 3 garlic cloves, minced

- 1 tablespoon ginger, grated

- 1 tablespoon curry powder

- 1 teaspoon ground cumin

- 1 teaspoon ground coriander

- 1/2 teaspoon turmeric

- 1/4 teaspoon cayenne pepper (optional, for heat)

- 1 can diced tomatoes

- 1 can coconut milk

- 2 cups vegetable broth

- 2 cups cauliflower florets

- 2 tablespoons coconut oil

- Salt and pepper to taste

- Fresh cilantro for garnish

For the Cauliflower Rice:

- 1 medium-sized cauliflower head

- 2 tablespoons olive oil

- Salt and pepper to taste

Instructions:

1. To make the Lentil Curry, heat coconut oil in a large pot over medium heat. Add diced onion and cook until softened, about 5 minutes.

2. Add minced garlic and grated ginger to the pot and cook for another 2 minutes, until fragrant.

3. Add curry powder, cumin, coriander, turmeric, and cayenne pepper (if using) to the pot. Stir well to coat the onion mixture with the spices.

4. Pour in the can of diced tomatoes, coconut milk, and vegetable broth. Stir to combine all the ingredients.

5. Add the rinsed red lentils to the pot and bring the mixture to a simmer. Let it cook for about 20-25 minutes, or until the lentils are tender.

6. While the lentils are cooking, prepare the cauliflower rice. Cut the cauliflower head into florets and place them in a food processor. Pulse until the cauliflower resembles rice-like grains.

7. Heat olive oil in a large skillet over medium heat. Add the cauliflower rice and sauté for 5-7 minutes, until it becomes tender. Season with salt and pepper.

8. Once the lentils are cooked, add the cauliflower florets to the pot. Stir gently to incorporate them into the curry.

9. Allow the curry to simmer for another 5-10 minutes, until the cauliflower is tender but still has a slight bite to it.

10. Taste the curry and adjust the seasoning with salt and pepper as desired.

11. Serve the Lentil Curry over a bed of cauliflower rice and garnish with fresh cilantro.

12. Enjoy your flavorful and healthy Lentil Curry with Cauliflower Rice!

This recipe is not only delicious but also versatile. You can customize it by adding vegetables like spinach, bell peppers, or peas to the curry, or topping it with a dollop of yogurt for extra creaminess. The options are endless, so don't be afraid to get creative and make it your own.

Baked Teriyaki Salmon with Steamed Vegetables Recipe

Ingredients:

- 2 salmon fillets

- ½ cup soy sauce

- ¼ cup honey

- 2 tablespoons rice vinegar

- 1 tablespoon minced garlic

- 1 tablespoon minced ginger

- 1 teaspoon sesame oil

- Two cups of mixed veggies, including snap peas, carrots, and broccoli

- 1 tablespoon sesame seeds (optional)

- Salt and pepper to taste

Instructions:

1. Adjust the oven temperature to 400°F (200°C) and place parchment paper on a baking pan.

2. In a small bowl, whisk together the soy sauce, honey, rice vinegar, minced garlic, minced ginger, and sesame oil to make the teriyaki sauce.

3. Place the salmon fillets on the prepared baking sheet and season with salt and pepper.

4. Pour half of the teriyaki sauce over the salmon fillets, ensuring they are evenly coated.

5. Bake the salmon in the preheated oven for 12-15 minutes or until the fish is cooked through and flakes easily with a fork.

6. While the salmon is cooking, steam the mixed vegetables until they are tender, but still slightly crisp. You can use a steamer basket on the stove or microwave-safe container with a little water.

7. Once the salmon is done, remove it from the oven and set aside to rest for a few minutes.

8. In a small saucepan, heat the remaining teriyaki sauce over medium heat until it thickens slightly.

9. Arrange the steamed vegetables on a serving plate and place the baked teriyaki salmon fillets on top.

10. Drizzle the thickened teriyaki sauce over the salmon and vegetables.

11. Sprinkle sesame seeds on top for garnish, if desired.

12. Serve the baked teriyaki salmon with steamed vegetables immediately and enjoy!

Note: You can serve this dish with steamed rice or noodles for a more satisfying meal. You can also add other favorite vegetables or modify the teriyaki sauce ingredients to suit your taste.

CHAPTER 6

6.1 Crispy baked kale chips

Crispy Baked Kale Chips Recipe

Ingredients:

- 1 bunch of kale

- 2 tablespoons of olive oil

- 1 teaspoon of salt

- Optional toppings: garlic powder, Parmesan cheese, smoked paprika, nutritional yeast

Instructions:

1. Preheat your oven to 350°F (175°C).

2. Wash the kale thoroughly and ensure it is completely dry. To dry it off, you may either use a salad spinner or a fresh kitchen towel.

3. Cut off the kale leaves' rough stalks. Tear the kale leaves into bite-sized pieces and place them in a large mixing bowl.

4. Drizzle the olive oil over the torn kale leaves. Massage the oil into the leaves using your hands, ensuring that each piece is coated.

5. Sprinkle salt evenly over the kale leaves. You can also add any optional toppings at this point, such as garlic powder, Parmesan cheese, smoked paprika, or nutritional yeast. Adapt the quantity to your personal taste preferences.

6. Toss the kale leaves gently to evenly distribute the oil, salt, and toppings.

7. Line a baking sheet with parchment paper or foil for easy cleanup. Spread the kale leaves in a single layer on the baking sheet, ensuring they are not overlapping.

8. Place the baking sheet in the preheated oven and bake for 10-15 minutes, or until the kale leaves are crispy and lightly browned. Keep an eye on the

chips during the last few minutes of baking to prevent them from burning.

9. Once the kale chips are done, remove them from the oven and let them cool on the baking sheet for a few minutes. As they cool, they will get increasingly crispier.

10. Serve the crispy baked kale chips immediately as a healthy snack or side dish. Enjoy!

Note: Make sure to store any leftover kale chips in an airtight container to maintain their crispiness. It's preferable to consume them within a few days.

6.2 Hummus and veggie platter

Hummus and Veggie Platter Recipe

If you're looking for a healthy and delicious appetizer or snack, a hummus and veggie platter is the perfect choice. Made with homemade hummus and a variety of fresh, colorful vegetables, this recipe is not only easy to prepare but also packed with nutrients. Here's a simple recipe to create a flavorful and visually appealing hummus and veggie platter.

Ingredients:

For the Hummus:

- 1 can (15 oz) of chickpeas, drained and rinsed

- 2 garlic cloves, minced

- 3 tablespoons of tahini

- 3 tablespoons of lemon juice

- 2 tablespoons of olive oil

- 1/2 teaspoon of cumin

- Salt and pepper to taste

- Water (as needed for desired consistency)

For the Veggie Platter:

- Carrot sticks

- Celery sticks

- Cucumber slices

- Bell pepper strips (assorted colors)

- Cherry tomatoes

- Radishes (sliced)

- Broccoli florets

- Cauliflower florets

Instructions:

1. Start by making the hummus. In a food processor or blender, combine the chickpeas, garlic, tahini, lemon juice, olive oil, cumin, salt, and pepper. Blend until smooth.

2. If the mixture is too thick, gradually add water, 1 tablespoon at a time, until desired consistency is reached. Continue blending until well combined.

3. After tasting the hummus, taste again and adjust the ingredients to your taste. You can add more tahini, lemon juice, or spices if desired.

4. Spoon the hummus into a serving bowl and lightly coat with olive oil. You can also sprinkle

some paprika or fresh herbs on top for added flavor and presentation.

5. Prepare the vegetables by washing and cutting them into bite-sized pieces. Arrange them on a large platter or individual serving plates.

6. Place the bowl of hummus in the center of the platter or next to the vegetables.

7. Serve the hummus with the variety of fresh vegetables, allowing guests to dip and enjoy.

Tips:

- Go ahead and use your imagination while choosing your vegetables. You can add other vegetables such as sugar snap peas, zucchini strips, or radicchio leaves to the platter.

- If you want to make this recipe even more colorful, use a mix of different colored bell peppers and cherry tomatoes.

- You can also garnish the platter with fresh herbs like parsley, cilantro, or dill for added freshness and flavor.

- Serve the hummus and veggie platter with some pita bread or whole-grain crackers for a more substantial snack or appetizer option.

- If you have any leftover hummus, store it in an airtight container in the refrigerator for up to a week. It makes a tasty spread for sandwiches or a dip for other veggies or chips.

Whether you're hosting a party or simply want a healthy snack option, this hummus and veggie platter is a crowd-pleaser. The creamy and flavorful hummus pairs perfectly with the crisp and vibrant assortment of vegetables. Enjoy this nutritious and delicious appetizer that is sure to satisfy your taste buds.

Recipe for Stuffed Bell Peppers with Black Beans and Quinoa

Ingredients:

- 4 large bell peppers (any color)

- 1 cup cooked quinoa

- 1 cup canned black beans, rinsed and drained

- 1 small onion, diced

- 2 cloves garlic, minced

- 1 cup diced tomatoes

- One cup of shredded cheese, either Mexican blend or cheddar

- 1 tablespoon olive oil

- 1 teaspoon ground cumin

- 1/2 teaspoon chili powder

- Salt and pepper to taste

- Fresh cilantro, for garnish

Instructions:

1. Preheat your oven to 375°F (190°C). Grease a baking dish lightly or line it with parchment paper.

2. Prepare the bell peppers by slicing off their tops, removing the seeds, and hollowing out the insides. Ensure the peppers can stand upright on their own. Put them in the baking dish that has been prepared.

3. Heat the olive oil in a big skillet over medium heat.

 Add the diced onion and minced garlic, sautéing for about 3-4 minutes until they become translucent.

4. Add the cooked quinoa, black beans, diced tomatoes, cumin, chili powder, salt, and pepper to the skillet. Stir everything together and cook for an additional 2-3 minutes to allow the flavors to blend.

5. Spoon the quinoa and black bean mixture into each bell pepper until they are filled. Press down gently to ensure they are tightly packed.

6. Bake the baking dish for thirty minutes in a preheated oven covered with aluminum foil.

7. After 30 minutes, remove the foil and sprinkle the shredded cheese on top of each stuffed bell pepper. Return them to the oven for an additional 10-15 minutes or until the cheese is melted and bubbly.

8. Once cooked, remove the stuffed bell peppers from the oven and let them cool slightly. Garnish with fresh cilantro and serve hot.

These stuffed bell peppers with quinoa and black beans are a delicious and healthy vegetarian meal option. They are a filling and healthy option because they are high in protein, fiber, and flavor.

CHAPTER 7

Sweet treats without the guilt

7.1 Dark chocolate and almond energy bites

Dark Chocolate and Almond Energy Bites Recipe

Ingredients:

- 1 cup pitted dates

- 1 cup almonds

- 1/2 cup dark chocolate chips

- 1 tablespoon chia seeds

- 1 tablespoon honey

- 1 tablespoon cocoa powder

- 1/2 teaspoon vanilla extract

- Pinch of salt

Instructions:

1. In a food processor, add the pitted dates and almonds. Process until thoroughly blended and finely chopped.

2. Add the dark chocolate chips, chia seeds, honey, cocoa powder, vanilla extract, and salt to the food processor. Process until all the ingredients are fully mixed and sticking together.

3. Take tablespoon-sized portions of the mixture and roll them into small balls using your hands. Arrange the energy balls on a parchment paper-lined baking sheet.

4. Once all the mixture is rolled into balls, refrigerate them for at least 30 minutes to firm up.

5. Store the dark chocolate and almond energy bites in an airtight container in the refrigerator for up to two weeks.

These energy bites are perfect for a quick and healthy snack on-the-go. They provide a good balance of protein, healthy fats, and natural sugars from the dates. The dark chocolate chips add a touch of indulgence, while the almonds add a satisfying crunch. The chia seeds and cocoa powder provide an extra boost of nutrients.

Not only are these energy bites delicious, but they are also packed with nutritional benefits. Dark chocolate is rich in antioxidants and can help improve heart health. Almonds are a great source of protein, healthy fats, and vitamin E. Chia seeds are high in fiber and omega-3 fatty acids, which are essential for brain health.

Whether you need a pick-me-up during the day or a pre-workout snack, these dark chocolate and almond energy bites will give you the sustained energy you need. They are easy to make and can be customized to your liking by adding other ingredients like coconut flakes, peanut butter, or dried fruits.

So, next time you're in need of a healthy and satisfying snack, give this dark chocolate and almond energy bites recipe a try.

7.2 Banana-oatmeal cookies

Banana-Oatmeal Cookies Recipe:

Ingredients:

- 2 ripe bananas

- 1 cup rolled oats

- 1/2 cup peanut butter (or any nut or seed butter of your choice)

- 1/4 cup honey or maple syrup

- 1/4 cup raisins or any other dried fruits (optional)

- 1/4 cup chopped nuts (optional)

- 1/2 teaspoon vanilla extract

- 1/2 teaspoon cinnamon

- 1/4 teaspoon salt

Instructions:

1. Preheat your oven to 350°F (175°C) and line a baking sheet with parchment paper.

2. In a medium-sized bowl, mash the bananas until smooth.

3. Add the peanut butter, honey or maple syrup, vanilla extract, cinnamon, and salt to the banana mixture. Stir until well combined.

4. Gradually add the rolled oats to the wet mixture, stirring well after each addition. If desired, fold in the raisins or chopped nuts.

5 Spoonful of the dough should be dropped, separated by roughly 2 inches, onto the baking sheet that has been prepared.

6. Flatten each cookie slightly with the back of a spoon.

7. Bake for 12-15 minutes, until the edges are golden brown and the cookies are set in the center.

8. Remove from the oven and let cool on the baking sheet for a few minutes, then transfer to a wire rack to cool completely.

9. Enjoy your delicious and healthy banana-oatmeal cookies!

These cookies are a great option for a nutritious snack or breakfast on the go. They are naturally sweetened with bananas and honey or maple syrup, and packed with fiber from the rolled oats. The peanut butter adds a creamy and nutty flavor, but feel-free to use any nut or seed butter of your choice.

You can also customize these cookies by adding your favorite mix-ins, such as raisins, dried fruits, or chopped nuts. They are easy to make and perfect for using up ripe bananas. Give these Banana-Oatmeal Cookies a try and enjoy a tasty treat.

7.3 Berry chia pudding

Berry Chia Pudding Recipe

Ingredients:

- One cup of mixed berries, comprising raspberries, blueberries, and strawberries

- 1/4 cup chia seeds

- 1 cup almond milk (or any non-dairy milk)

- One tablespoon of maple syrup (or your preferred sweetener)

- 1/2 teaspoon vanilla extract

- A pinch of salt

Instructions:

1. In a blender or food processor, blend the mixed berries until smooth.

2. In a medium-sized bowl, combine the blended berries, chia seeds, almond milk, maple syrup, vanilla extract, and salt. Stir well to ensure the chia seeds are fully coated.

3. Cover the bowl and place it in the refrigerator for at least 4 hours or overnight. By doing this, the

liquid will be absorbed by the chia seeds, giving the dish a pudding-like consistency.

4. After the chia pudding has set, give it a good stir to evenly distribute the seeds and berries.

5. Serve the Berry Chia Pudding in bowls or glass jars and top with additional berries, nuts, or granola if desired.

6. Enjoy immediately, or store in the refrigerator for up to 3 days.

Note: You can customize this recipe by using different types of milk, such as coconut milk or cashew milk, and by adding your favorite toppings like shredded coconut, cacao nibs, or sliced almonds. Try different things and make them uniquely yours! This recipe serves 2-3 people but can easily be doubled or halved depending on your needs. Whether enjoyed as a healthy breakfast or a delicious dessert, this Berry Chia Pudding is sure to satisfy your cravings and provide you with a nutritious and filling treat

CHAPTER 8

Beverages for hydration and blood sugar control

8.1 Green smoothie with spinach and avocado

Green Smoothie with Spinach and Avocado Recipe

Ingredients:

- 2 cups fresh spinach leaves

- 1 ripe avocado, peeled and pitted

- 1 medium banana

- One cup of normal or coconut water

- 1 tablespoon honey or maple syrup (optional)

- Juice of 1 lime

- Ice cubes (optional)

Instructions:

1. In a blender, combine the spinach, avocado, banana, coconut water, honey (if using), and lime juice.

2. Process the mixture at a high speed until it's creamy and smooth.

3. If desired, add a few ice cubes to make the smoothie colder and frothier.

4. Continue blending until the ice cubes are fully incorporated.

5. Taste the smoothie and adjust the sweetness by adding more honey or maple syrup if needed.

6. Immediately serve the smoothie by pouring it into glasses.

Optional Additions:

- 1 tablespoon chia seeds, for added fiber and omega-3 fatty acids

- 1 scoop of protein powder, for a boost of protein

- 1 tablespoon flaxseed oil, for a dose of healthy fats

Additional Notes:

- This recipe is for a basic green smoothie, but feel free to modify it to suit your preferences. You can add other fruits such as apples, pears, or mangoes for a different flavor profile.

- If you don't have coconut water, you can use regular water or any other liquid of your choice, such as almond milk or coconut milk.

- The addition of sweetener is optional, as the banana and honey or maple syrup already provide natural sweetness. Adjust according to your taste preference.

- This smoothie is best enjoyed fresh, but you can store any leftovers in an airtight container in the refrigerator for up to 24 hours. Give it a quick blend before serving again.

Enjoy this nutritious and delicious green smoothie as a refreshing drink or as a healthy breakfast option. It's packed with vitamins, minerals, and antioxidants from the spinach and avocado to support your overall well-being.

8.2 Cucumber and mint infused water

Cucumber and Mint Infused Water Recipe

Ingredients:

- 1 medium cucumber

- 10-12 fresh mint leaves

- 1 liter of water

- Ice cubes (optional)

Instructions:

1. Give the cucumber a good wash to get rid of any residue or debris. Slice it into thin rounds or dice it into small pieces, depending on your preference.

2. Take the fresh mint leaves and gently crush them with your hands to release their oils and flavors. This will help enhance the taste of the infused water.

3. In a large pitcher or glass jar, add the sliced cucumber and crushed mint leaves.

4. Pour the water over the cucumber and mint. If desired, you can also add a few ice cubes to make the water refreshingly chilled.

5. Stir the ingredients gently to combine and allow the flavors to infuse. You can use a long spoon or a clean utensil for this.

6. Let the cucumber and mint infused water sit in the refrigerator for at least one hour, or overnight if you prefer a more intense flavor.

7. Once the water has infused to your liking, you can strain out the solids or simply leave them in the water if you enjoy the added texture.

8. Serve the cucumber and mint infused water in glasses with additional ice cubes, if desired. You can also garnish each glass with a sprig of fresh mint for an extra touch of elegance.

9. Enjoy your refreshing and hydrating cucumber and mint infused water! This drink is perfect for staying hydrated on a hot summer day or for adding a burst of flavor to your daily water intake. It's a healthy and delicious alternative to sugary beverages.

Tips:

- Experiment with the cucumber and mint ratio to find your preferred flavor. You can add more cucumber for a more pronounced freshness, or more mint for a stronger herbal taste.

- If you prefer sweeter infused water, you can add a small amount of honey or a few drops of stevia to the mixture. Stir well to dissolve the sweetener.

- Feel free to get creative with other additions to your cucumber and mint infused water. You can add lemon slices, lime wedges, or even a few berries for additional flavor and nutrients.

Remember to stay hydrated and enjoy the rejuvenating benefits of this simple and refreshing cucumber and mint infused water recipe.

8.3 Healing turmeric golden milk

Turmeric Golden Milk has been used for centuries in Ayurvedic medicine as a natural remedy for a wide range of health issues. This healing drink is made with turmeric, a powerful anti-inflammatory spice that is high in antioxidants and has been shown to provide numerous health benefits. The addition of other warm spices like cinnamon and ginger, along with a touch of sweetness from honey or maple syrup, makes this drink not only delicious but also soothing and comforting.

To make Turmeric Golden Milk, you will need the following ingredients:

- One cup of non-dairy milk, such as almond milk.

- 1 teaspoon of ground turmeric

- 1/2 teaspoon of ground cinnamon

- 1/4 teaspoon of ground ginger

- 1 tablespoon of honey or maple syrup (optional for sweetness)

- A pinch of black pepper (this helps to increase the bioavailability of the turmeric)

- A sprinkle of ground nutmeg (optional for additional flavor)

Here are the steps to prepare this healing drink:

1. In a small saucepan, heat the almond milk over medium heat until it becomes warm but not boiling.

2. Add the ground turmeric, cinnamon, ginger, and black pepper to the warm milk. Whisk well until all the spices are fully incorporated and there are no lumps.

3. Continue to heat the mixture for about 5 minutes, stirring occasionally to prevent burning.

4. Turn off the heat source and let the mixture cool a little.

5. If desired, add honey or maple syrup to sweeten the drink. Until the sweetener is completely dissolved, stir thoroughly.

6. Pour the Turmeric Golden Milk into a mug and sprinkle a dash of ground nutmeg on top for an extra touch of flavor.

7. Enjoy your healing Turmeric Golden Milk while it's warm. The warm spices and soothing properties of turmeric will help to calm your body and mind, providing a sense of relaxation and well-being.

It's important to note that turmeric can stain, so be cautious when handling it and ensure you clean any utensils or surfaces that come into contact with the spice.

Turmeric Golden Milk can be enjoyed at any time of the day, but many people find it especially beneficial to consume before bed to promote a restful night's sleep. So sit back, relax, and savor the delicious, healing goodness of Turmeric Golden Milk.

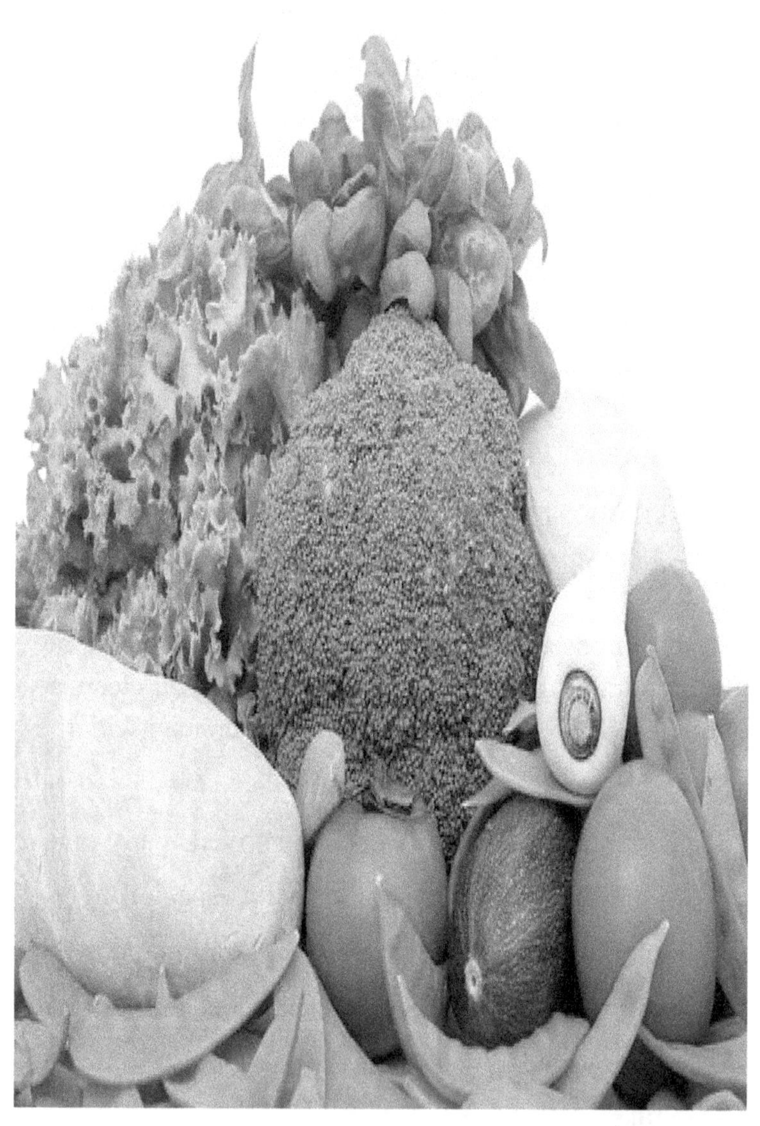

CHAPTER 9

Tips and tricks for success

9.1 How to shop for diabetic-friendly plant-based foods

Managing diabetes can be challenging, but a plant-based diet can help maintain blood sugar levels and overall health. If you have diabetes and are looking to incorporate more plant-based foods into your diet, here are some tips on how to shop for diabetic-friendly plant-based foods.

1. Focus on whole, unprocessed foods: Choose whole plant-based foods that are minimally processed. Instead of relying on packaged foods, opt for fresh fruits, vegetables, whole grains, legumes, nuts, and seeds.

2. Choose low glycemic index (GI) foods: The glycemic index ranks foods based on how they affect blood sugar levels. Foods with a low GI are beneficial for diabetics as they cause a slower rise in blood sugar levels. Some examples of low GI plant-based foods include non-starchy vegetables, whole grains like quinoa and barley, legumes like lentils and chickpeas, and most fruits.

3. Read food labels carefully: When purchasing packaged plant-based foods, carefully read the labels to identify any added sugars, unhealthy fats, and artificial ingredients. Look for foods with minimal added sugars and avoid products with high amounts of unhealthy fats like trans fats or hydrogenated oils.

4. Focus on nutrient density: Choose plant-based foods that are rich in nutrients. Opt for foods like leafy greens, cruciferous vegetables, berries, nuts, and seeds, as they are packed with vitamins, minerals, and antioxidants. These nutrient-dense foods can help support overall health and well-being, especially for those with diabetes.

5. Include a variety of protein sources: Plant-based proteins can be an excellent addition to a diabetic-friendly diet. Opt for protein sources like tofu, tempeh, edamame, lentils, chickpeas, and quinoa. These options provide essential amino acids, fiber, and are lower in saturated fat compared to animal-based proteins.

6. Avoid added sugars and sweeteners: Be cautious of hidden sugars in plant-based food products. Many plant-based products, such as dairy alternatives and snacks, may contain added sugars. Choose unsweetened or naturally sweetened options instead. Look for natural sweeteners like stevia, monk fruit, or use small amounts of non-nutritive sweeteners like erythritol or xylitol if needed.

7. Plan and prep your meals: Before heading to the grocery store, plan out your meals for the week. Having a meal plan can help you make a shopping list that includes all the necessary ingredients. Preparing meals at home allows you to control the ingredients and portion sizes, making it easier to manage your blood sugar levels.

8. Shop the perimeter of the grocery store: When shopping, focus on the outer aisles of the grocery store, where fresh produce, whole grains, and plant-based proteins are typically located. These are generally healthier options than heavily processed foods found in the center aisles.

9. Experiment with new foods: Trying new plant-based foods and recipes can keep your meals interesting and prevent boredom. Explore different fruits, vegetables, grains, and plant-based proteins to find the ones you enjoy the most. Incorporate a variety of flavors, textures, and colors into your meals to ensure a well-balanced diet.

10. Consult a registered dietitian: If you're uncertain about making dietary changes or need personalized guidance in managing your diabetes, consider consulting a registered dietitian who specializes in plant-based diets. They can help you create a meal plan that meets your individual needs and provide ongoing support.

Remember; always consult with your healthcare provider before making any significant changes to your diet, especially if you have diabetes. By shopping for diabetic-friendly plant-based foods and incorporating them into your meals, you can take control of your health and manage your diabetes effectively.

9.2 Dining out strategies for type 2 diabetics

Dining out can be challenging for individuals with Type 2 diabetes, as it may lead to unhealthy food choices and difficulties in managing blood sugar levels. However, with a few strategies in place, dining out can still be enjoyable while maintaining a balanced diet. Here are some tips and strategies for dining out for Type 2 diabetics:

1. Plan Ahead: Before heading out, it is crucial to plan your meal in advance. Many restaurants nowadays have their menus available online, allowing you to review and decide on healthier options ahead of time. Look for dishes that are lower in carbohydrates, saturated fats, and added sugars.

2. Choose the Right Restaurant: Selecting a restaurant that offers a variety of healthy options can make a significant difference. Look for venues that focus on fresh ingredients, whole foods, and offer lighter meals. Additionally, ethnic restaurants like Mediterranean or Middle Eastern tend to have diabetic-friendly choices such as grilled or baked proteins, vegetables, and whole grains.

3. Practice Portion Control: Be aware of portion sizes when dining out, as they are often larger than what you would consume at home. Consider sharing a meal with a friend or ask for a take-out box to portion out half of your meal before you start eating. This way, you can enjoy your favorite dishes while managing your portion sizes.

4. Modify Your Order: Don't be afraid to ask for modifications to suit your dietary needs. Requesting grilled or baked options instead of fried, swapping starchy sides for vegetables or salads, and asking for sauces or dressings on the side can help you control your carbohydrate and calorie intake.

5. Be Mindful of Hidden Sugars: Be cautious of hidden sugars in sauces, dressings, and condiments. Ask for sugar-free or low-sugar alternatives or ask if they can provide these items on the side, so you can control how much you consume.

6. Watch Your Beverage Choices: Sugary beverages like soda, sweetened iced tea, or fruit juices can quickly raise blood sugar levels. Opt for water, unsweetened tea or coffee, or choose sugar-free options instead. Also, be mindful of alcoholic beverages as they can affect blood sugar levels. If you choose to drink alcohol, do so in moderation and accompany it with food.

7. Don't Skip Meals: If you know you'll be dining out later in the day, don't skip meals leading up to it. This can cause you to overeat and make less healthy choices. Instead, maintain your regular meal routine and consider having a smaller, balanced meal earlier in the day to help control your appetite and blood sugar levels.

8. Be Prepared with Snacks: If you anticipate long wait times or delays in getting your food at the restaurant, have a healthy snack on hand to prevent low blood sugar. Choose snacks that are high in protein and fiber, such as nuts, Greek yogurt, or cut-up vegetables with hummus.

9. Stay Active: Incorporate some physical activity into your day, especially before dining out. Taking a walk or engaging in light exercise can help lower blood sugar levels and improve insulin sensitivity.

10. Monitor Blood Sugar Levels: It's essential to monitor your blood sugar levels before and after dining out. This will help you understand the impact of different foods on your body and adjust your diet and lifestyle accordingly.

Remember, dining out should be an enjoyable experience, even for individuals with Type 2 diabetes. By planning ahead, making mindful choices, and listening to your body's needs, you can manage your blood sugar levels while still savoring delicious meals at your favorite restaurants.

9.3 Managing stress and emotional eating

Managing Stress and Emotional Eating

Stress and emotional eating often go hand in hand, as many people turn to food as a way to cope with stress and emotions. Unfortunately, this can lead to a cycle of unhealthy eating habits and weight gain. However, with some strategies and techniques, it is possible to manage stress and emotional eating effectively.

1. Identify triggers: The first step in managing stress and emotional eating is to identify the triggers that lead to it. It could be certain events, situations, or emotions that prompt you to reach for food. By becoming aware of these triggers, you can start to find healthier ways to cope with them.

2. Develop healthy coping mechanisms: Instead of turning to food when stressed or emotional, it is important to find alternative coping mechanisms. Engaging in activities such as exercise, deep breathing, meditation, or finding a hobby can help distract from the urge to eat. These activities can also help to reduce stress and promote emotional well-being.

3. Practice mindful eating: Mindful eating is a technique that involves paying attention to the present moment while eating, focusing on the taste, texture, and smell of the food. By being more present during meals, you can better tune into your body's hunger and fullness cues, which can help prevent overeating and emotional eating. Take time to savor your food, chew slowly, and really engage with the experience of eating.

4. Keep a food journal: A food journal can help you track your eating habits and identify patterns or triggers for emotional eating. Note down your eating schedule, what you consume, and your emotional state. This can help you become more aware of your emotional eating patterns and allow you to make healthier choices in the future.

5. Build a support system: Having a strong support system can be beneficial in managing stress and emotional eating. Reach out to friends, family, or a therapist to talk about your feelings and emotions. They can provide guidance, encouragement, and accountability. Remember, you are not alone in this struggle, and seeking support can make a big difference.

6. Plan and prepare meals in advance: When stress and emotions run high, it's easy to resort to convenience foods or unhealthy snacks. By planning and preparing meals in advance, you can ensure that you have nutritious options readily available. This can help prevent impulsive and emotional food choices.

7. Prioritize self-care: Taking care of your overall well-being is essential in managing stress and emotional eating. Prioritize getting enough sleep, engaging in regular physical activity, and finding activities that bring you joy and relaxation. Self-care activities like taking a bath, reading a book, or practicing mindfulness can help reduce stress and improve your mood, making you less likely to turn to food for comfort.

8. Seek professional help if needed: If you find that stress and emotional eating are significantly impacting your life and well-being, don't hesitate to seek professional help. A therapist or registered dietitian can provide guidance and support tailored to your specific needs and helps you develop healthy coping mechanisms.

Remember that managing stress and emotional eating is a journey, and it may take time to break old habits and develop new ones. Along the journey, remind yourself to be kind to yourself and have patience. With time and effort, you can learn to manage stress in healthier ways and establish a positive relationship with food.

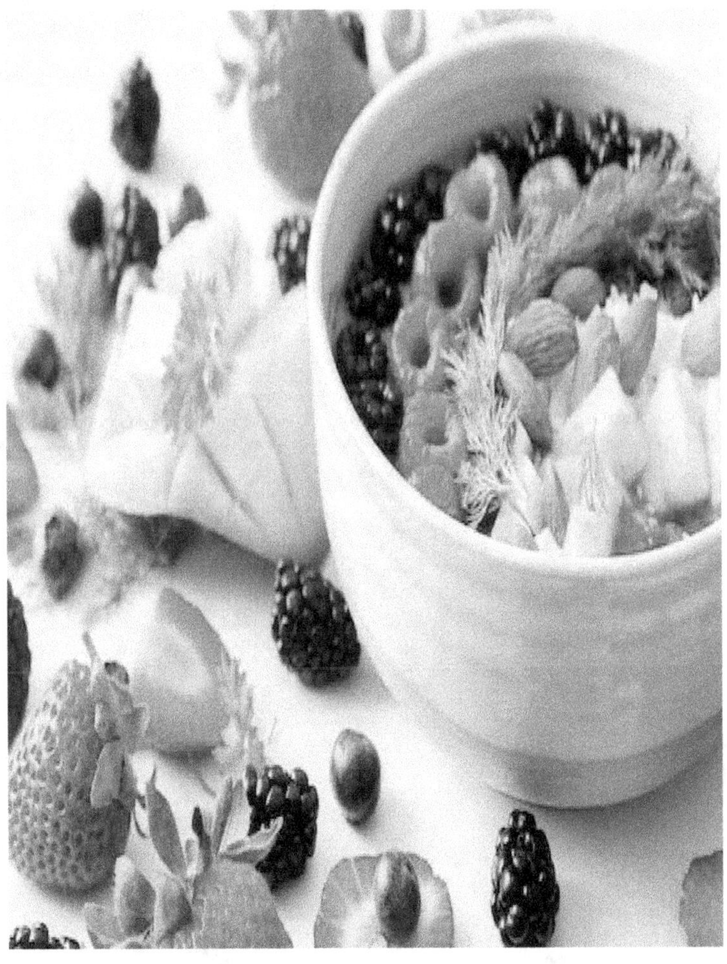

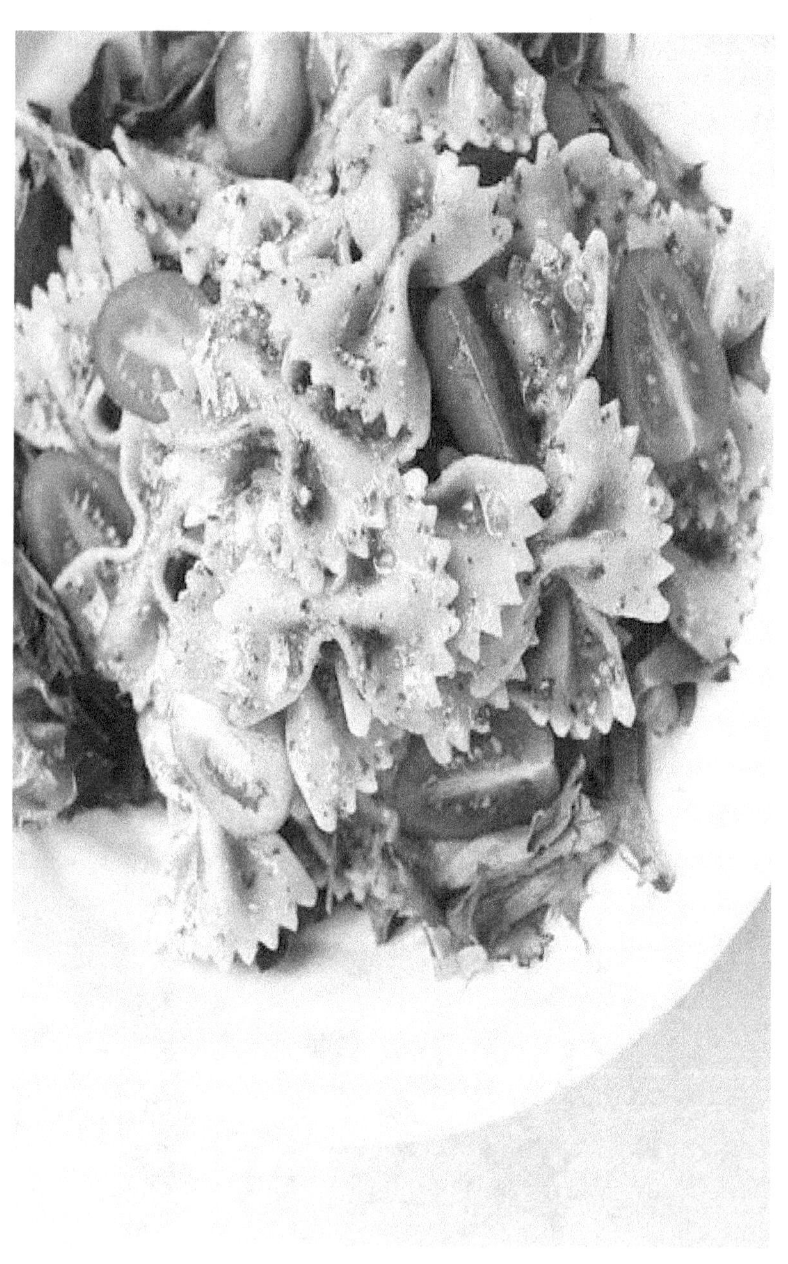

CHAPTER 10

10.1 One-week meal plan for type 2 diabetics

Monday:

- **Breakfast:** 1 scrambled egg with spinach and mushrooms, 1 slice of whole grain toast, and a small apple.

- **Lunch:** Grilled chicken breast with steamed broccoli and quinoa.

- **Snack:** 1 ounce of almonds.

- **Dinner:** Baked salmon with roasted Brussels sprouts and a side salad with mixed greens, tomatoes, and cucumbers.

- **Dessert:** Sugar-free yogurt with berries.

Tuesday:

- **Breakfast:** Overnight oats made with ½ cup rolled oats, 1 cup unsweetened almond milk, 1 tablespoon chia seeds, and ½ cup mixed berries.

- **Lunch:** Turkey lettuce wrap with sliced turkey breast, lettuce, tomato, cucumber, and mustard.

- **Snack:** Celery sticks with 2 tablespoons of natural peanut butter.

- **Dinner:** Stir-fried tofu with mixed vegetables (broccoli, bell peppers, carrots) served over brown rice.

- **Dessert:** Sliced melon.

Wednesday:

- **Breakfast:** Vegetable omelet with bell peppers, onions, and mushrooms, served with a side of whole grain toast.

- **Lunch:** Quinoa salad with cherry tomatoes, cucumber, feta cheese, and lemon vinaigrette.

- **Snack:** Greek yogurt with cinnamon.

- **Dinner:** Steamed asparagus, roasted sweet potatoes, and grilled chicken breast.

- **Dessert:** Sugar-free jello.

Thursday:

- **Breakfast**: 1 slice of whole grain toast with avocado and a poached egg.

- **Lunch:** Spinach salad with grilled shrimp, cherry tomatoes, cucumbers, and balsamic vinaigrette.

- **Snack:** Carrot and celery sticks with hummus.

- **Dinner:** Steamed green beans and baked cod served with quinoa on the side.

- **Dessert:** Dark chocolate square.

Friday:

- **Breakfast:** Veggie scrambles with bell peppers, onions, spinach, and feta cheese.

- **Lunch:** Grilled chicken salad with mixed greens, strawberries, almonds, and a light vinaigrette.

- **Snack:** 1 ounce of walnuts.

- **Dinner:** Turkey meatballs with zucchini noodles and marinara sauce.

- **Dessert:** Sugar-free popsicle.

Saturday:

- **Breakfast:** Greek yogurt with sliced banana and a sprinkle of granola.

- **Lunch:** A mixed green salad with lentil soup.

- **Snack:** Hard-boiled egg.

- **Dinner:** Grilled salmon with roasted cauliflower and a side of quinoa.

- **Dessert:** Berries topped with a whipped cream dollop.

Sunday:

- **Breakfast:** Whole grain pancakes with sugar-free syrup and a small serving of fruit.

- **Lunch:** Turkey and vegetable wrap with whole wheat tortilla, lettuce, tomato, cucumber, and mustard.

- **Snack:** Sugar-free yogurt with a sprinkle of granola.

- **Dinner:** Grilled chicken with roasted sweet potatoes and steamed broccoli.

- **Dessert**: Dark chocolate-covered strawberries.

It's important to note that every individual's dietary needs may vary, so it's recommended to consult with a healthcare professional or a registered dietitian who can provide personalized guidance for managing type 2 diabetes.

10.2 Grocery list for healthy plant-based eating

1. Fresh fruits and vegetables: Include a variety of colors such as leafy greens, berries, tomatoes, cucumbers, carrots, bell peppers, etc.

2. Whole grains: Choose options like brown rice, quinoa, oats, whole wheat pasta, whole grain bread, etc.

3. Legumes: Stock up on beans, lentils, chickpeas, and tofu. These are excellent sources of protein and fiber.

4. Nuts and seeds: Include almonds, walnuts, chia seeds, flax seeds, etc. These provide healthy fats, protein, and additional nutrients.

5. Plant-based milk: Opt for almond milk, oat milk, soy milk, or any other non-dairy alternative.

6. Healthy fats: Add avocados, olive oil, coconut oil, and nut butter to your list. These are excellent providers of important fatty acids.

7. Herbs and spices: Keep a variety of herbs and spices like garlic, turmeric, ginger, basil, oregano, etc. to add flavor to your dishes.

8. Non-dairy yogurt: Choose plain or flavored options made from coconut, almond, or soy.

9. Plant-based protein sources: Look for meat alternatives like tempeh, seitan, tofu, and other plant-based proteins like edamame, quinoa, and buckwheat.

10. Plant-based condiments: Include items like hummus, salsa, tahini, nutritional yeast, and mustard for added flavor.

11. Plant-based snacks: Stock up on whole food snacks like rice cakes, popcorn, nuts, dried fruits, and energy bars.

12. Healthy beverages: Don't forget to add water, herbal teas, and green tea to your list. These are great options for hydration and antioxidants.

13. Frozen fruits and vegetables: Keep a selection of frozen fruits and vegetables on hand for quick and convenient meals and smoothies.

14. Dark chocolate: Consider adding a small amount of dark chocolate (70% or higher cocoa content) to your list for a healthy indulgence.

15. Meal prep staples: Include items like vegetable broth, canned tomatoes, whole grain bread, and other pantry staples for easy meal preparation.

16. Fresh herbs and greens: Consider growing your own herbs and salad greens at home to ensure a supply of fresh ingredients.

17. Seaweed: Add dried seaweed or sea vegetables to your list for added minerals and flavor in your meals.

18. Healthy sweeteners: Look for options like maple syrup, agave nectar, or stevia as healthier alternatives to refined sugar.

19. Fermented foods: Consider including items like sauerkraut, kimchi, or kombucha for their probiotic benefits.

20. Sustainability-conscious choices: If possible, choose organic, locally sourced, and sustainably produced options to support your health and the health of the planet.

Remember to plan your meals in advance and consider the recipes you'll be making to ensure you have all the necessary ingredients on your grocery list. Happy and healthy plant-based eating!

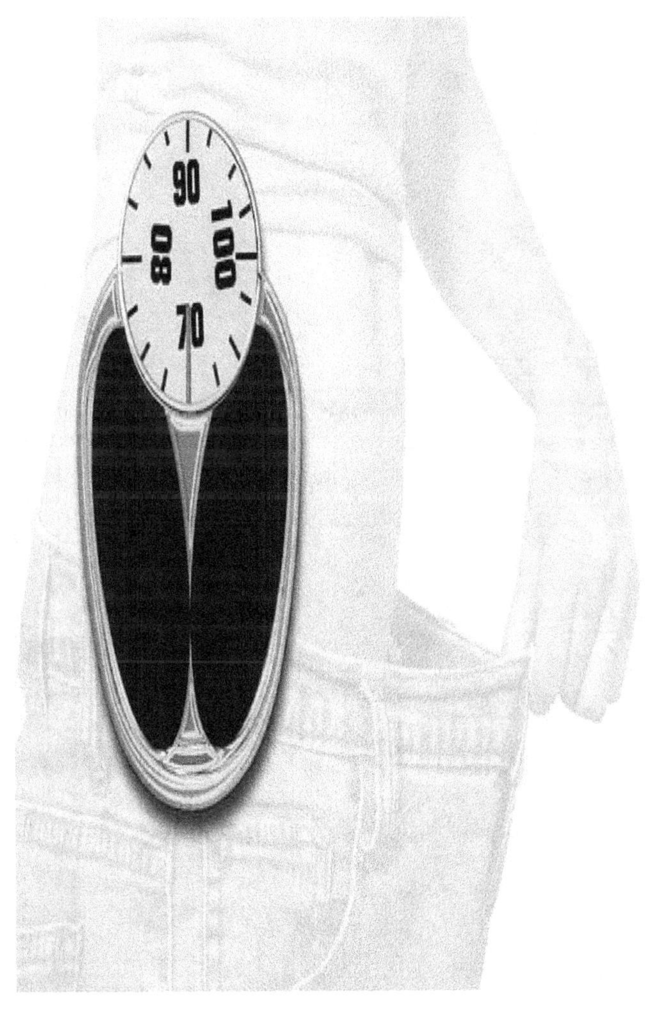

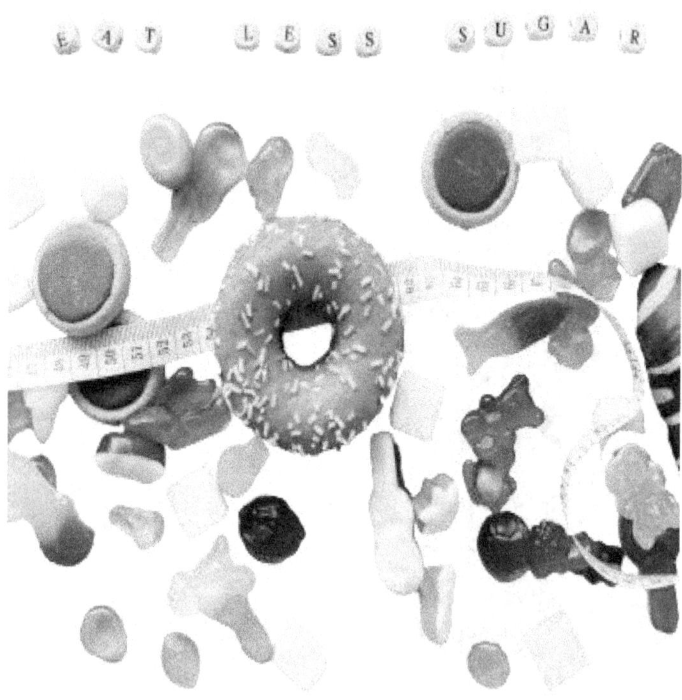
EAT LESS SUGAR

CONCLUSION

In conclusion, type 2 diabetic plant-based diet cookbooks are an incredible resource for individuals looking to improve their health and manage their condition effectively. These cookbooks offer a wide array of delicious and nutritious recipes that prioritize whole foods, plant-based ingredients, and mindful cooking techniques.

By adopting a plant-based diet, individuals with type 2 diabetes can experience numerous benefits. These cookbooks emphasize the consumption of fruits, vegetables, whole grains, legumes, nuts, and seeds, all of which are rich in essential nutrients, fiber, and antioxidants. This type of dietary approach has been associated with improved blood sugar control, weight management, heart health, and overall well-being.

Furthermore, plant-based diets can also help reduce the risk of developing other chronic diseases commonly associated with type 2 diabetes, such as cardiovascular disease and certain types of cancer.

By focusing on plant-based ingredients, individuals can minimize their intake of saturated and trans fats, cholesterol, and processed foods, which are often contributors to these health issues.

Type 2 diabetic plant-based diet cookbooks not only provide an extensive collection of recipes but also offer guidance on meal planning, portion control, and smart substitutions for traditional ingredients. These resources are invaluable for individuals who may be new to plant-based eating or are unsure of how to incorporate a variety of flavors and ingredients into their meals.

Moreover, these cookbooks emphasize the importance of mindful eating and paying attention to hunger and fullness cues. They encourage individuals to savor each bite, engage with the cooking process, and create a positive relationship with food. This mindfulness can lead to healthier eating habits, improved portion control, and a more enjoyable dining experience.

Another significant advantage of type 2 diabetic plant-based diet cookbooks is their versatility. They cater to individuals with different dietary preferences and restrictions, as they often offer options for gluten-free, dairy-free, and soy-free recipes. This inclusivity ensures that everyone can find delicious and suitable recipes that align with their specific needs.

Furthermore, the inclusion of nutritional information for each recipe is a crucial aspect of these cookbooks. People with type 2 diabetes often need to monitor their carbohydrate intake, and these cookbooks provide clear information about the nutritional content of each dish. This allows individuals to make informed choices and maintain better control over their blood sugar levels.

Additionally, these cookbooks also provide tips for meal prepping and batch cooking, enabling individuals to save time and have healthy options readily available throughout the week. This can be especially beneficial for those with busy schedules or limited access to fresh ingredients. By planning and preparing meals in advance, individuals can ensure they have nutritious, balanced meals on hand, reducing the temptation to rely on less healthy options.

Type 2 diabetic plant-based diet cookbooks not only offer practical advice on cooking and meal planning but also promote a more sustainable and environmentally friendly way of eating. By reducing reliance on animal products, individuals can decrease their carbon footprint and contribute to a healthier planet for future generations.

Lastly, type 2 diabetic plant-based diet cookbooks provide a wealth of information, delicious recipes, and practical guidance for individuals looking to manage their condition through healthy eating. By following the principles outlined in these cookbooks, individuals can enhance their overall health, reduce the risk of developing complications, and discover a more enjoyable and flavorful approach to managing their type 2 diabetes.

Embracing a plant-based lifestyle not only benefits individuals on a personal level but also holds the potential to positively impact global health and the environment. With the support and guidance of these cookbooks, individuals with type 2 diabetes can embark on a journey towards improved health, better blood sugar control, and a more vibrant and fulfilling life.